Pocket Atlas of Cranial
Magnetic Resonance Imaging

Second Edition

Pocket Atlas of Cranial Magnetic Resonance Imaging

Second Edition

Scott W. Atlas, M.D.

Professor of Radiology
Chief, Neuroradiology
Stanford University Medical Center
Stanford, California

Richard T. Kaplan, M.D.

Clinical Assistant Professor of Radiology
Stanford University Medical Center
Stanford, California

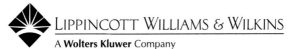

LIPPINCOTT WILLIAMS & WILKINS
A **Wolters Kluwer** Company

Philadelphia · Baltimore · New York · London
Buenos Aires · Hong Kong · Sydney · Tokyo

Acquisitions Editor: Joyce-Rachel John
Developmental Editor: Murray E. Hill
Production Editor: Allison L. Risko
Manufacturing Manager: Tim Reynolds
Cover Designer: Patricia Gast
Compositor: LWW Desktop Division, NY
Printer: Sheriden Press

Printed in the USA

Library of Congress Cataloging-in-Publication Data
Atlas, Scott W., 1955–
    Pocket atlas of cranial magnetic resonance imaging / Scott W. Atlas, Richard T. Kaplan.
       p. ; cm.
    Includes bibliographical references and index.
    ISBN 0-7817-3573-4 (alk. paper)
    1. Brain—Magnetic resonance imaging—Atlases. 2. Brain—Magnetic resonance
imaging—Handbooks, manuals, etc. I. Kaplan, Richard T. II. Title.
    [DNLM: 1. Brain—anatomy & histology—Atlases. 2. Brain—anatomy &
histology—Handbooks. 3. Anatomy, Cross-Sectional—Atlases. 4. Anatomy,
Cross-Sectional—Handbooks. 5. Magnetic Resonance Imaging—Atlases. 6. Magnetic
Resonance Imaging—Handbooks. WL 17 A8803p 2001]
    RC386.6.M34 A85 2001
    616.8′047548—dc21
                                                                                    2001029908

Care has been taken to confirm the accuracy of the information presented and to describe generally accepted practices. However, the authors, editors, and publisher are not responsible for errors or omissions or for any consequences from application of the information in this book and make no warranty, expressed or implied, with respect to the currency, completeness, or accuracy of the contents of the publication. Application of this information in a particular situation remains the professional responsibility of the practitioner.

The authors, editors, and publisher have exerted every effort to ensure that drug selection and dosage set forth in this text are in accordance with current recommendations and practice at the time of publication. However, in view of ongoing research, changes in government regulations, and the constant flow of information relating to drug therapy and drug reactions, the reader is urged to check the package insert for each drug for any change in indications and dosage and for added warnings and precautions. This is particularly important when the recommended agent is a new or infrequently employed drug.

Some drugs and medical devices presented in this publication have Food and Drug Administration (FDA) clearance for limited use in restricted research settings. It is the responsibility of the health care provider to ascertain the FDA status of each drug or device planned for use in their clinical practice.

10 9 8 7 6 5 4 3 2 1

Preface

This book was designed to provide a pocket atlas of anatomy for anyone interested in cranial magnetic resonance (MR) imaging. This includes all physicians involved with the neurosciences, as well as fellows, residents, and medical students who are interpreting brain MR studies or learning cerebral neuroanatomy. MR technologists will also find the information in this book helpful.

Images in the sagittal, axial and coronal plane are included to assist in understanding the anatomy. For each labeled image, numbered arrows identify an anatomic structure. A corresponding legend is placed on the same page. A localizer image is also included to indicate the imaging plane and location.

All of the images in this book were acquired on a General Electric 1.5-T Signa LX MR scanner. The technical parameters utilized for each pulse sequence are as follows. Fast spin echo T2-weighted axial and coronal brain images: TR/TE/excitations = 4000/100/2, slice thickness = 5mm, interslice gap = 1mm, FOV = 24 X 24, matrix 256 X 256. Spin echo T1-weighted sagittal brain images: TR/TE/excitations = 500/18/1, slice thickness = 5mm, interslice gap = 2mm, FOV = 24 X 24, matrix 256 X 192. Spin echo T1-weighted high-resolution sella images: TR/TE/excitations = 500/18/5, slice thickness = 3mm, interslice gap = 0.3mm, FOV = 16 X 16, matrix 256 X 224. 3D Time of flight circle of Willis images: TR/TE/excitations = 34/min/1, slice thickness = 1mm, FOV = 24 X 24, matrix 512 X 128.

Acknowledgments

Special thanks to Kevin Woolley for his contribution to this project.

TPIS

Contents

Sagittal Brain 1
Axial Brain 7
Coronal Brain 23
Sella Images 47
Intracranial MRA 55
References 62
Index 63

Sagittal Brain _____

Sagittal Brain

1. temporal lobe
2. sylvian fissure
3. frontal lobe
4. parietal lobe
5. occipital lobe
6. tentorium
7. cerebellum

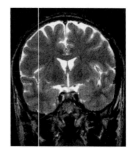

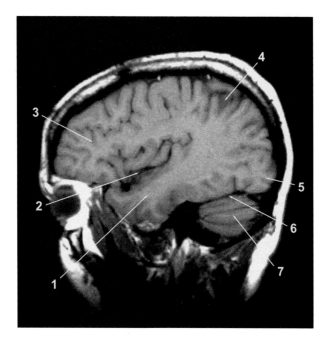

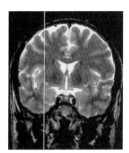

1. temporal lobe
2. temporal horn lateral ventricle
3. inferior frontal gyrus
4. atrium lateral ventricle
5. hippocampus

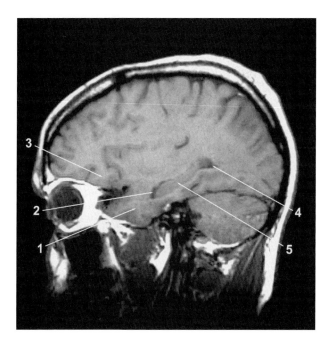

Sagittal Brain

1. head caudate nucleus
2. body lateral ventricle
3. thalamus
4. pulvinar
5. parietoccipital sulcus
6. calcarine sulcus
7. middle cerebellar peduncle
8. pons
9. midbrain

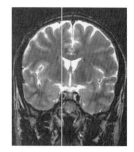

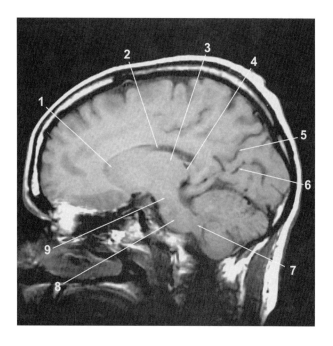

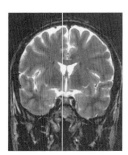

1. prepontine cistern
2. cingulate sulcus
3. thalamus
4. fornix
5. precuneus
6. parietooccipital sulcus
7. anterior calcarine sulcus
8. inferior colliculus
9. primary fissure
10. tuber
11. fourth ventricle
12. cerebellar tonsil

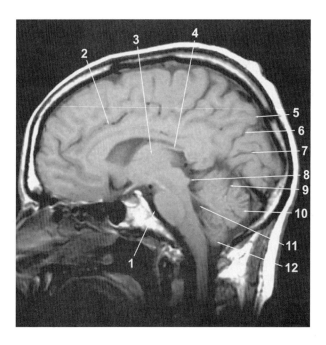

1. pituitary gland
2. genu corpus callosum
3. septum pellucidum
4. fornix
5. splenium corpus callosum
6. vein of Galen
7. superior sagittal sinus
8. straight sinus
9. quadrigeminal plate
10. cerebral aqueduct
11. midbrain decussation
12. medulla
13. pons

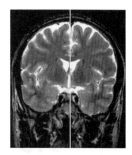

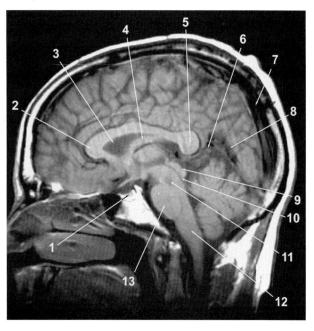

Axial Brain _____

1. vertebral artery
2. medulla
3. foramen of Luschka
4. cerebellar tonsil

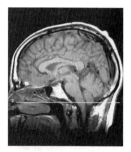

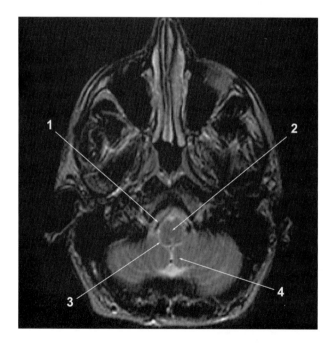

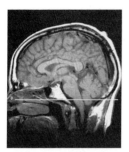

1. medullary pyramid
2. clivus
3. inferior medullary olive
4. post-olivary sulcus
5. cerebellar hemisphere
6. cisterna magna
7. inferior cerebellar peduncle

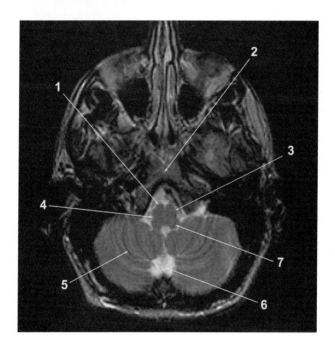

1. basilar artery
2. sphenoid bone
3. anterior inferior cerebellar artery
4. flocculus
5. inferior cerebellar peduncle
6. foramen of Luschka

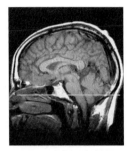

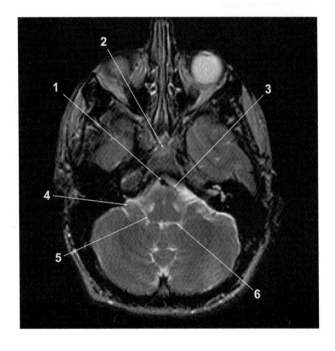

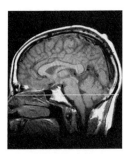

1. basilar artery
2. pons
3. facial colliculus
4. Meckel's cave
5. fourth ventricle
6. dentate nucleus
7. uvula
8. nodulus
9. middle cerebellar peduncle
10. flocculus
11. trigeminal nerve in
    cerebellopontine angle cistern

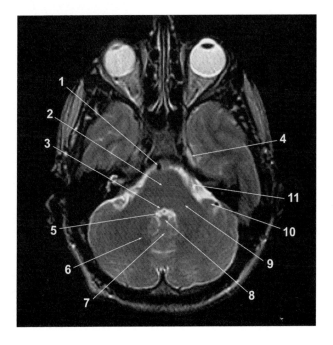

1. cavernous internal carotid artery
2. pons
3. superior limb, cerebellopontine fissure
4. fourth ventricle
5. superior cerebellar peduncle
6. transverse sinus
7. prepontine cistern
8. dorsum sella
9. temporal lobe

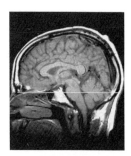

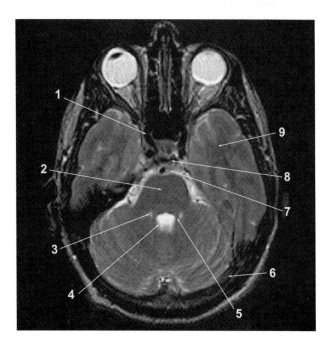

1. optic canal
2. anterior clinoid process
3. temporal horn
4. infundibulum
5. superior cerebellar artery
6. inferior colliculus
7. ambient cistern
8. superior cerebellar vermis

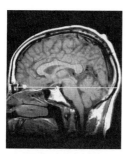

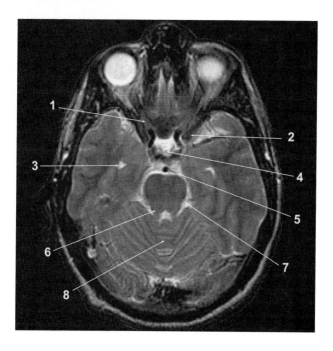

1. cerebral peduncle
2. M1 segment, middle cerebral artery
3. gyrus rectus
4. optic chiasm
5. optic tract
6. uncus
7. posterior cerebral artery
8. interpeduncular cistern
9. occipital pole
10. torcular herophili
11. cerebellar vermis

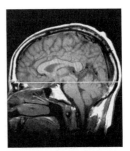

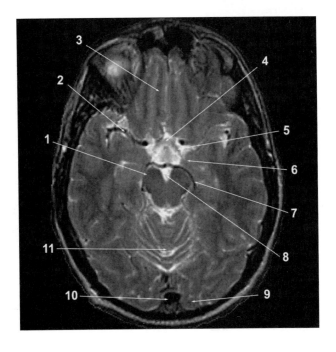

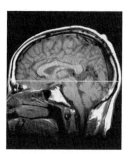

1. orbital sulcus
2. optic tract
3. mammillary body
4. substantia nigra
5. hippocampus
6. periaqueductal gray matter
7. superior colliculus
8. superior cerebellar vermis
9. quadrigeminal plate cistern
10. red nucleus
11. cerebral peduncle

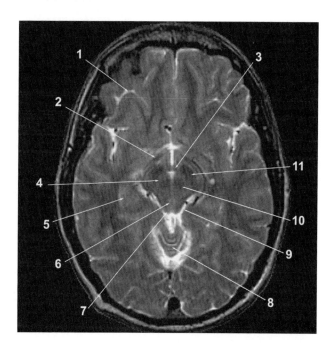

1. anterior commissure
2. fornix
3. third ventricle
4. posterior commissure
5. putamen
6. globus pallidus
7. thalamus
8. hippocampus tail
9. sagittal sinus

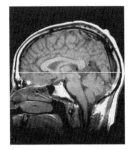

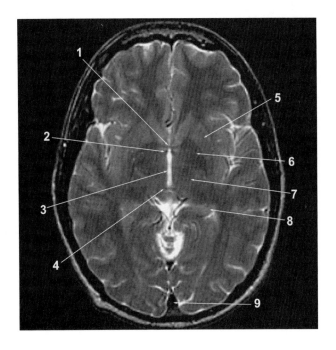

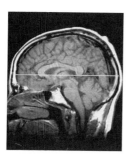

1. anterior limb, internal capsule
2. putamen
3. insula
4. middle cerebral artery branches in sylvian fissure
5. posterior limb, internal capsule
6. head, caudate nucleus
7. external capsule
8. genu, internal capsule
9. foramen of Monro
10. thalamus
11. atrium, lateral ventricle
12. calcar avis
13. calcarine sulcus

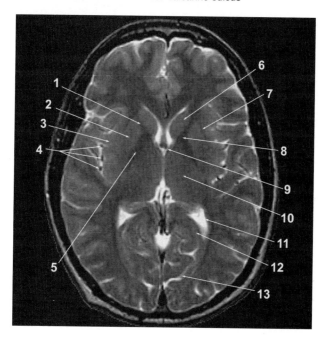

1. septum pellucidum
2. genu, of corpus callosum
3. frontal horn, lateral ventricle
4. putamen
5. splenium, of corpus callosum
6. straight sinus
7. tail, caudate nucleus

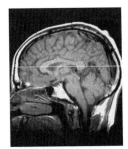

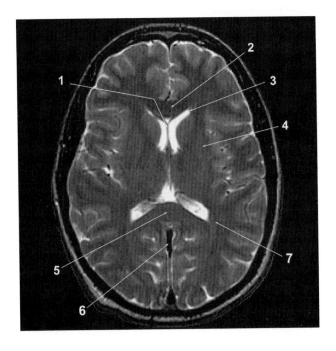

1. superior sagittal sinus
2. corona radiata
3. horizontal portion, sylvian fissure
4. parietooccipital sulcus
5. genu corpus callosum
6. body/head caudate nucleus
7. body, lateral ventricle
8. fornix

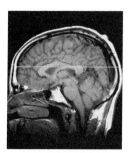

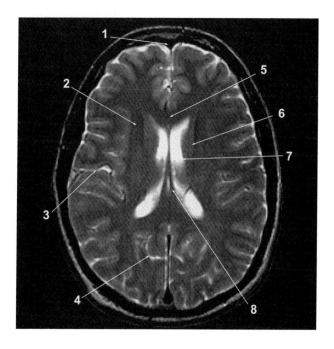

1. anterior cerebral artery
2. body, lateral ventricle
3. corona radiata
4. precentral sulcus
5. postcentral sulcus
6. superior sagittal sinus
7. body, corpus callosum

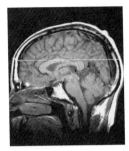

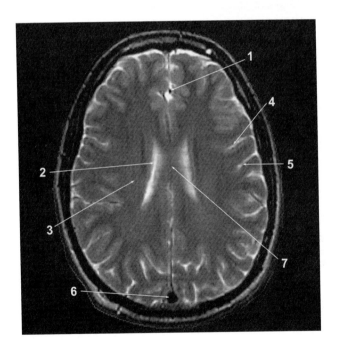

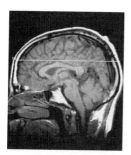

1. superior frontal sulcus
2. precentral sulcus
3. central gyrus
4. cingulate gyrus
5. centrum semiovale
6. superior sagittal sinus

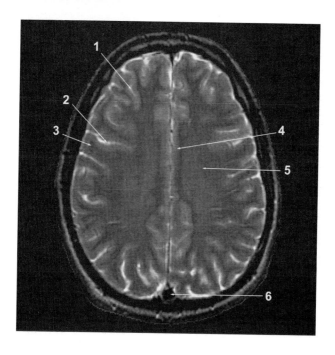

1. central sulcus
2. frontal white matter
3. superior sagittal sinus
4. interhemispheric fissure

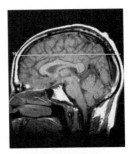

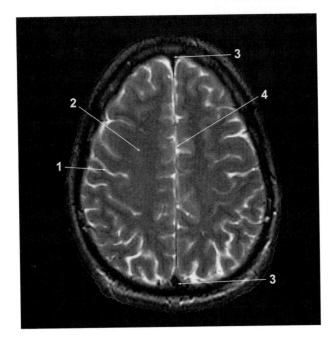

Coronal Brain _____

1. superior sagittal sinus
2. torcular herophili
3. transverse sinus

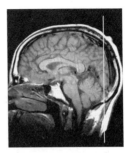

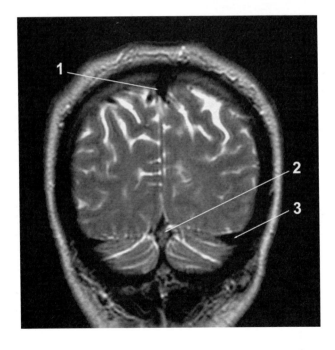

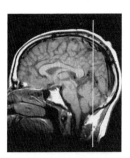

1. superior sagittal sinus
2. calcarine sulcus
3. tentorium cerebelli
4. parietooccipital sulcus
5. straight sinus
6. transverse sinus
7. cisterna magna

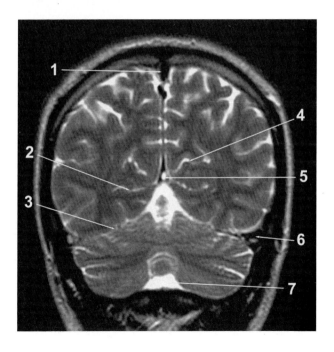

1. sigmoid sinus
2. superior cerebellar vermis
3. transverse sinus
4. cisterna magna

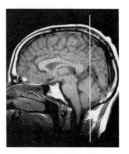

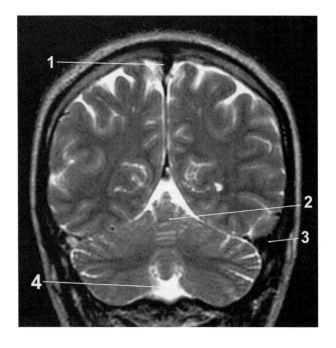

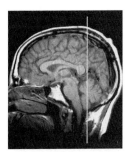

1. calcarine sulcus
2. superior sagittal sinus
3. straight sinus
4. occipital horn, lateral ventricle
5. transverse sinus
6. cerebellar white matter
7. dentate nucleus

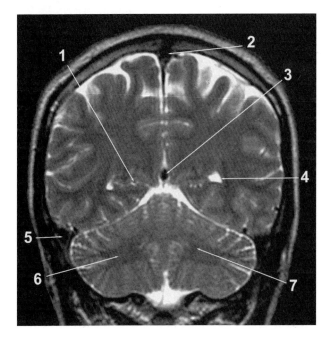

1. splenium, corpus callosum
2. posterior horn, lateral ventricle
3. calcarine sulcus
4. cerebellar tonsil
5. straight sinus
6. lingula
7. nodulus
8. uvula

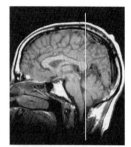

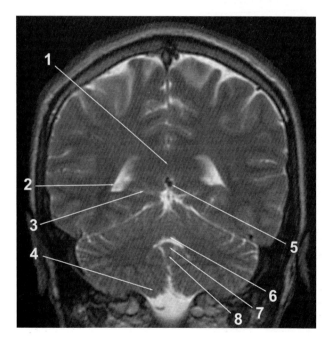

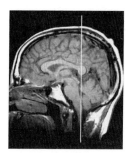

1. superior cerebellar peduncle
2. fourth ventricle
3. cerebellar tonsil
4. cingulate gyrus
5. splenium, corpus callosum
6. tentorium
7. horizontal fissure

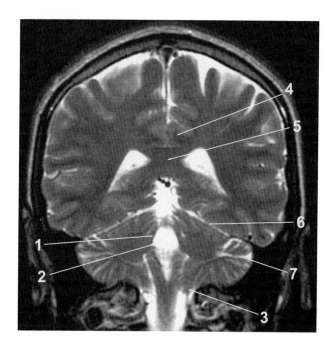

1. cerebral aqueduct
2. periaqueductal gray matter
3. middle cerebellar peduncle
4. medulla
5. fornix
6. vein of Galen
7. superior colliculus
8. inferior colliculus
9. superior cerebellar peduncle
10. cervical spinal cord

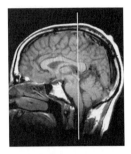

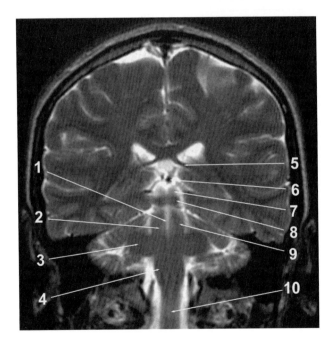

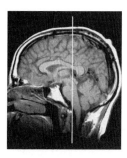

1. cingulate sulcus
2. cingulate gyrus
3. fornix
4. superior colliculus
5. temporal horn lateral ventricle
6. middle cerebellar peduncle
7. centrum semiovale
8. corona radiata
9. thalamus
10. hippocampus
11. trochlear nerve
12. medullary pyramid

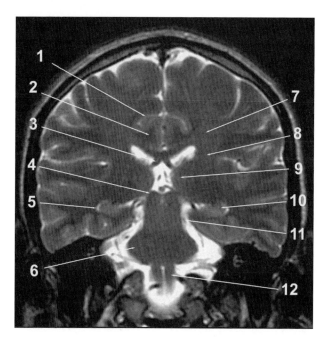

1. lateral geniculate body
2. parahippocampal gyrus
3. trigeminal nerve
4. vestibule
5. facial nerve
6. cochlear nerve
7. basal turn of cochlea
8. lateral semicircular canal
9. superior semicircular canal
10. pons
11. substantia nigra
12. third ventricle

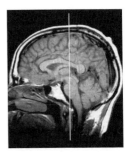

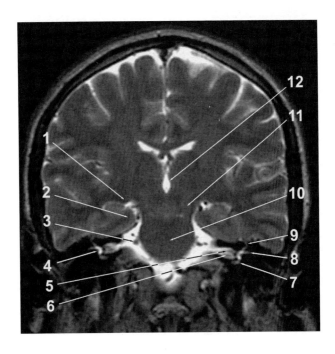

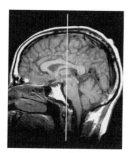

1. red nucleus
2. horizontal sylvian fissure
3. choroidal fissure
4. alveus
5. P2 segment, posterior cerebral artery
6. anterior inferior cerebellar artery
7. vertebral basilar junction
8. thalamus
9. subthalamic nucleus
10. interpeduncular cistern
11. occipitotemporal sulcus
12. trigeminal nerve

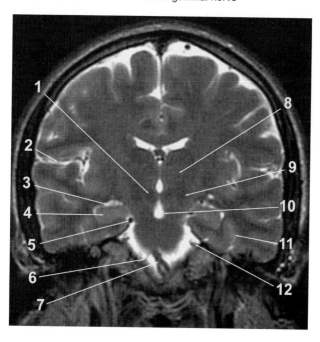

1. superior temporal gyrus
2. middle temporal gyrus
3. hippocampus
4. parahippocampal gyrus
5. basilar artery
6. body, corpus callosum
7. body, caudate nucleus
8. thalamus
9. optic tract
10. P1 segment, posterior cerebral artery
11. superior cerebellar artery
12. trigeminal nerve in Meckel's cave

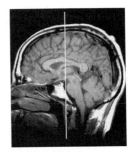

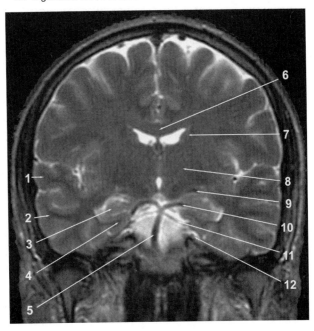

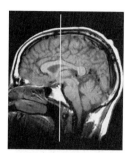

1. putamen
2. insular cortex
3. temporal horn lateral ventricle
4. body, corpus callosum
5. third ventricle
6. floor, third ventricle
   (hypothalamus)
7. amygdala

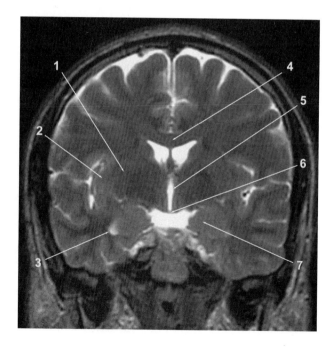

1. cingulate sulcus
2. septum pellucidum
3. body, caudate nucleus
4. putamen
5. horizontal segment, sylvian fissure
6. vertical segment sylvian fissure
7. uncinate fasciculus
8. globus pallidus
9. fornix

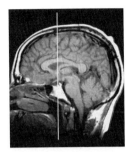

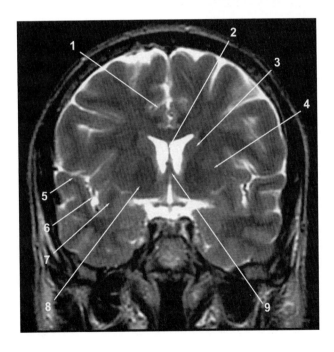

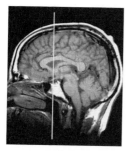

1. internal capsule
2. lentiform nucleus
3. A1 segment, anterior cerebral artery
4. supraclinoid internal carotid artery
5. optic chiasm
6. corona radiata
7. insular cortex
8. external capsule
9. M1 segment, middle cerebral artery
10. cavernous internal carotid artery
11. pituitary gland

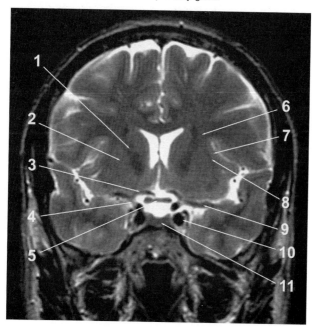

1. pericallosal artery
2. putamen
3. sylvian fissure
4. anterior commissure
5. superior sagittal sinus
6. falx cerebri
7. head, caudate nucleus
8. external capsule
9. rostrum, corpus callosum
10. prechiasmatic optic nerve

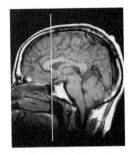

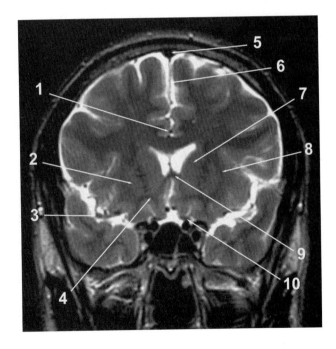

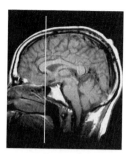

1. head, caudate nucleus
2. A2 segment, anterior cerebral artery
3. intracanalicular optic nerve
4. superior frontal gyrus
5. inferior frontal gyrus
6. frontal horn, lateral ventricle
7. temporal lobe

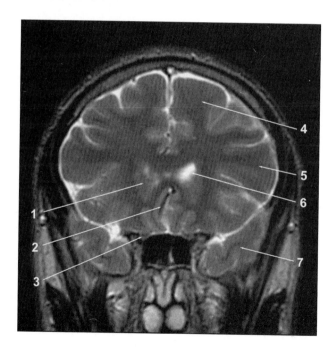

1. gyrus rectus
2. genu corpus callosum
3. interhemispheric fissure
4. superior frontal gyrus
5. middle frontal gyrus
6. inferior frontal gyrus
7. frontal horn lateral ventricle

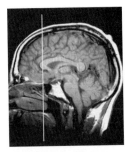

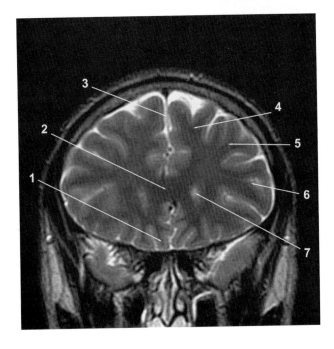

1. forceps minor
2. gyrus rectus
3. olfactory sulcus
4. medial orbital gyrus
5. pericallosal artery
6. superior sagittal sinus

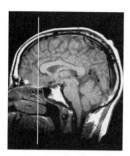

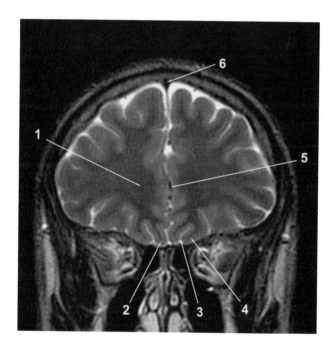

1. superior frontal sulcus
2. forceps minor
3. olfactory sulcus
4. olfactory tract
5. gyrus rectus
6. medial orbital gyrus
7. inferior frontal gyrus
8. cingulate gyrus
9. superior frontal gyrus

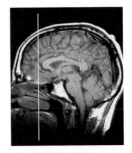

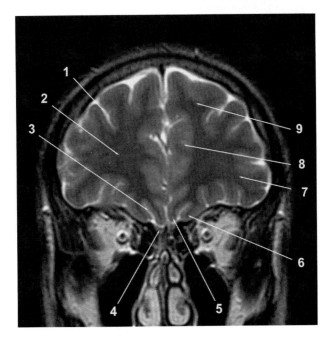

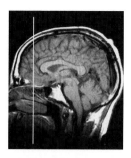

1. gyrus rectus
2. superior ophthalmic vein
3. perioptic cerebrospinal fluid
4. lateral rectus muscle
5. inferior rectus muscle
6. superior frontal gyrus
7. superior frontal sulcus
8. olfactory bulb
9. superior rectus muscle
10. superior oblique muscle
11. optic nerve
12. medial rectus muscle

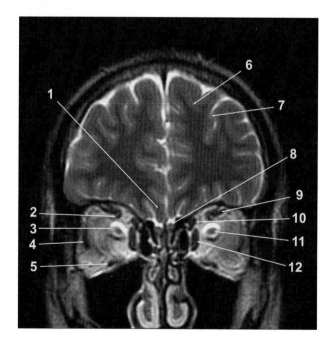

1. interhemispheric fissure
2. globe
3. medial orbital gyrus
4. superior sagittal sinus
5. superior frontal gyrus
6. inferior frontal gyrus

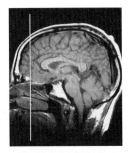

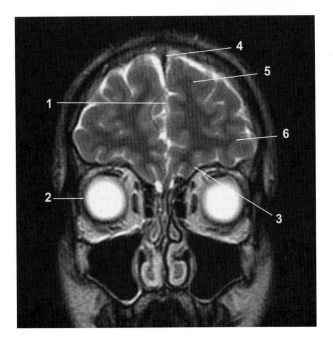

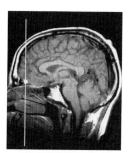

1. scalp
2. calvarium
3. cribriform plate

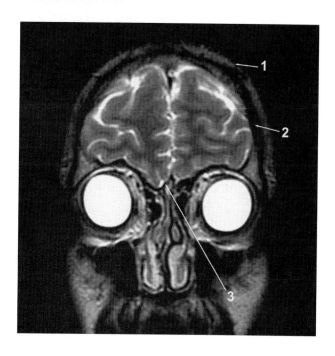

Sella Coronal _____

1. optic tract
2. suprasellar cistern
3. third ventricle
4. hypothalamus
5. Meckel's cave

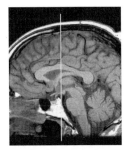

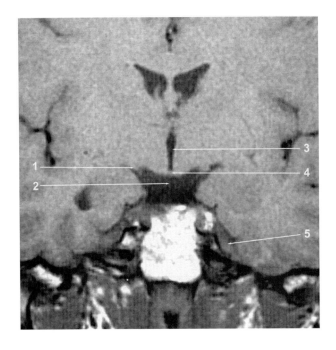

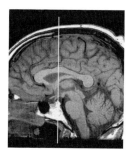

1. septum pellucidum
2. optic tract
3. dorsum sella
4. third ventricle
5. hypothalamus
6. oculomotor nerve
7. internal carotid artery

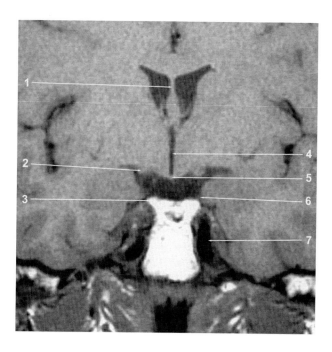

1. third ventricle
2. infundibulum
3. neurohypophysis
4. precavernous internal carotid artery
5. optic tract
6. oculomotor nerve
7. clivus
8. mandibular division trigeminal nerve

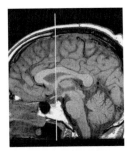

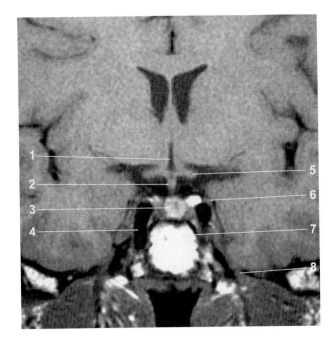

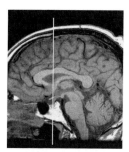

1. A1 segment, anterior cerebral artery
2. supraclinoid internal carotid artery
3. abducens nerve
4. maxillary division trigeminal nerve
5. suprachiasmatic recess
6. optic chiasm
7. M1 segment, middle cerebral artery
8. cavernous internal carotid artery
9. ophthalmic division trigeminal nerve
10. adenohypophysis

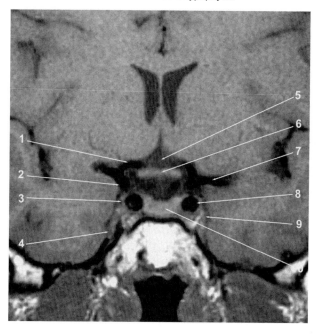

1. A2 segment anterior cerebral artery
2. cavernous internal carotid artery
3. ophthalmic division trigeminal nerve
4. optic tract
5. oculomotor nerve

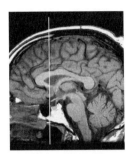

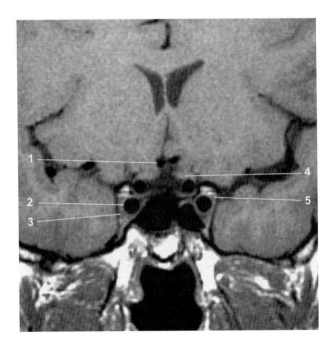

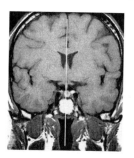

1. anterior commissure
2. infundibular recess
3. optic chiasm
4. infundibulum
5. adenohypophysis
6. posterior commissure
7. pineal gland
8. superior colliculus
9. inferior colliculus
10. cerebral aqueduct
11. mamillary body
12. hypothalamus
13. neurohypophysis

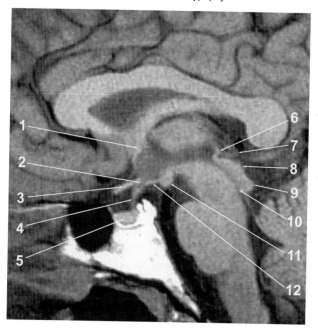

Intracranial MRA _____

1. M2 segment, middle cerebral artery
2. petrous segment, internal carotid artery
3. posterior cerebral artery
4. basilar artery
5. superior cerebellar artery
6. anterior communicating artery
7. middle cerebral artery branch in sylvian fissure
8. temporal branches of middle cerebral artery
9. cavernous internal carotid artery
10. A1 segment, anterior cerebral artery
11. A2 segment, anterior cerebral artery
12. ophthalmic artery
13. M1 segment, middle cerebral artery

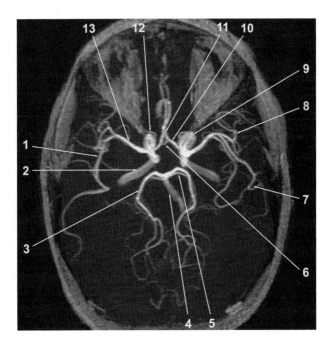

1. anterior communicating artery
2. A1 segment, anterior cerebral artery
3. cavernous internal carotid artery
4. supraclinoid internal carotid artery
5. genu, middle cerebral artery
6. temporal branches, middle cerebral artery
7. M2 segments, middle cerebral artery
8. middle cerebral artery branches in sylvian fissure
9. M1 segment, middle cerebral artery
10. A2 segment, middle cerebral artery

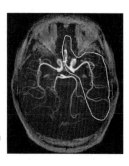

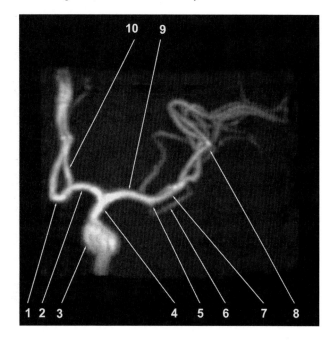

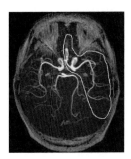

1. pericallosal artery
2. callosomarginal artery
3. A2 segment, anterior cerebral artery
4. supraclinoid internal carotid artery
5. cavernous internal carotid artery
6. frontal opercular branches, middle cerebral artery
7. M2 segment, middle cerebral artery

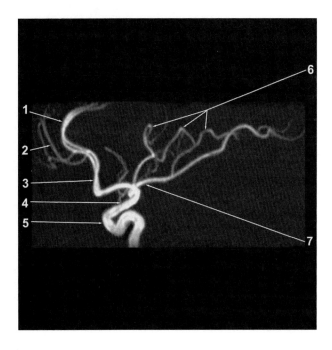

1. parietooccipital artery
2. temporal branches
3. superior cerebellar artery
4. basilar artery
5. vertebral artery
6. P1 segment, posterior cerebral artery
7. P2 segment, posterior cerebral artery
8. anterior inferior cerebellar artery

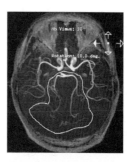

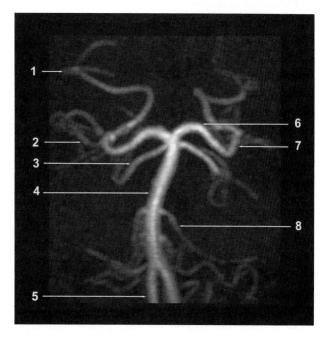

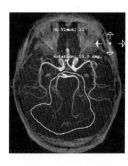

1. P1 segment, posterior cerebral artery
2. P2 segment, posterior cerebral artery
3. P3 segment, posterior cerebral artery
4. parietooccipital artery
5. calcarine artery
6. superior cerebellar artery
7. tonsillar loop, posterior inferior cerebellar artery
8. basilar artery

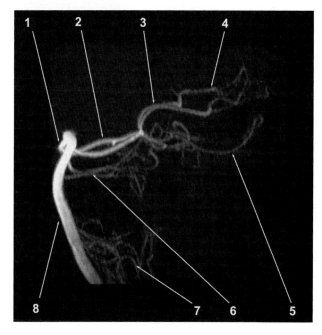

References

1. Atlas SW. *Magnetic resonance imaging of the brain and spine imaging*, 3rd ed. Philadelphia: Lippincott Williams & Wilkins, 2002 (in press).
2. Truwit CL, Lempert TE. *High resolution atlas of cranial neuroanatomy*. Baltimore: Williams and Wilkins, 1994.
3. Haughton VM, Daniels DL. *Pocket atlas of cranial magnetic resonance imaging*. New York: Raven Press, 1986.
4. DeArmond SJ, Fusco MM, Dewey MM. *Structure of the human brain: a photographic atlas*. New York: Oxford University Press, 1986.

Index

A

Abducens nerve, 51
Adenohypophysis, 51, 53
Alveus, 33
Ambient cistern, 13
Amygdala, 35
Anterior cerebral artery, 20
    A1 segment, 37, 51, 57, 58
    A2 segment, 52, 57, 59
Anterior commissure, 16, 38, 53
Anterior communicating artery,
    57, 58
Anterior inferior cerebellar
    artery, 10, 33, 60
Arteries. *See specific, e.g., Basilar*
    artery

B

Basilar artery, 10, 11, 34, 57, 60, 61

C

Calcar avis, 17
Calcarine artery, 61
Calcarine sulcus, 15, 17, 25, 27, 28
Callosomarginal artery, 59
Calvarium, 45
Carotid artery. *See* Internal
    carotid artery
Caudate nucleus
    body, 19, 34, 36
    head, 4, 17, 19, 38, 39
    tail, 18
Centrum semiovale, 21, 31

Cerebellar peduncle
    inferior 9, 10
    middle, 4, 11, 30, 31
    superior, 12, 29, 30
Cerebellar tonsil, 5, 8, 28, 29
Cerebellar vermis, 13, 14, 15
Cerebellar white matter, 27
Cerebellopontine fissure
    superior limb, 12
Cerebellum, 2
Cerebral aqueduct, 6, 30, 53
Cerebral peduncle, 14, 15
Cervical spinal cord, 30
Cingulate gyrus, 29, 31, 42
Cingulate sulcus, 5, 31, 36
Cistern. *See specific, e.g., Ambient*
    cistern
Cisterna magna, 9, 25, 26
Clinoid process
    anterior, 13
Clivus, 9, 50
Cochlea
    basal turn, 32
Cochlear nerve, 32
Colliculus
    inferior, 5, 13, 30, 53
    superior, 15, 30, 53
Commissure
    anterior, 16
    posterior, 16
Corona radiata, 19, 20, 31, 37
Corpus callosum
    body, 20, 34, 35
    genu, 6, 18, 19, 40
    rostrum, 38
    splenium, 6, 18, 28

Cribriform plate, 45

D

Dentate nucleus, 11, 27
Dorsum sella, 12, 49

E

External capsule, 17, 38

F

Facial colliculus, 11
Facial nerve, 32
Falx cerebri, 38
Flocculus, 10, 11
Foramen of Luschka, 8, 11
Foramen of Monro, 17
Forceps minor, 41, 42
Fornix, 5, 6, 16, 19, 30, 31, 36
Fourth ventricle, 5, 11, 12, 29
Frontal gyrus
    inferior, 39, 40, 42, 44
    middle, 40
    superior, 39, 40, 42, 43, 44
Frontal lobe, 2

G

Globe, 44
Globus pallidus, 16, 36
Gyrus
    cingulate, 21, 29, 31, 42
    frontal, 39, 40, 42, 43, 44
    medial orbital, 41, 42, 44
    parahippocampal, 32
    temporal, 34
Gyrus rectus, 14, 40, 41, 42, 43

H

Hippocampus, 3, 15, 16, 31, 34
Horizontal fissure, 29
Hypothalamus, 48, 49, 53

I

Inferior cerebellar peduncle, 9, 10
Inferior colliculus, 30, 53
Inferior rectus muscle, 43
Infundibular recess, 53
Infundibulum, 13, 50, 53
Insular cortex, 35, 37
Interhemispheric fissure, 22, 40, 44
Internal capsule, 17, 37
Internal carotid artery, 49
    cavernous, 12, 37, 51, 52, 57, 58, 59
    petrous segment, 57
    precavernous, 50
    supraclinoid, 37, 51, 58, 59
Interpeduncular cistern, 14, 33

L

Lateral geniculate body, 32
Lateral rectus muscle, 43
Lateral ventricle
    atrium, 3, 17
    body, 4, 19, 20
    frontal horn, 18, 39, 40
    occipital horn, 27
    posterior horn, 28
    temporal horn, 3, 13, 31, 35
Lentiform nucleus, 37
Lingula, 28

M

Mamillary body, 15, 53

Meckel's cave, 11, 34, 48
Medial orbital gyrus, 42, 44
Medial rectus muscle, 43
Medulla, 6, 8, 30
Medullary olive, 9
Medullary pyramid, 9, 31
Midbrain, 4
Midbrain decussation, 6
Middle cerebellar peduncle, 4
    10, 11, 30, 31
Middle cerebral artery, 14, 17,
    37, 51, 57, 58, 59

N

Neurohypophysis, 50, 53
Nodulus, 11, 28

O

Occipital lobe, 2
Occipital pole, 14
Oculomotor nerve, 49, 50, 52
Olfactory sulcus, 41, 42
Olfactory tract, 42
Olive
    inferior medullary, 9
Ophthalmic artery, 56
Ophthalmic vein, 43
Optic canal, 13
Optic chiasm, 14, 37, 51, 53
Optic nerve, 39, 38, 43
Optic tract, 14, 34, 48, 49, 50,
    52
Orbital sulcus, 15

P

Parahippocampal gyrus, 32
Parietal lobe, 2
Parietooccipital artery, 60, 61

Parietooccipital sulcus, 4, 5,
    19, 25
Periaqueductal gray matter,
    15, 30
Pericallosal artery, 38, 41, 58
Perioptic cerebrospinal fluid,
    43
Pineal gland, 53
Pituitary gland, 6, 38
Pons, 4, 6, 11, 12, 32
Posterior cerebral artery, 14,
    56
    P1 segment, 34, 60, 61
    P2 segment, 33, 60, 61
    P3 segment, 61
Posterior commissure, 16, 53
Posterior inferior cerebellar
    artery, 61
Precuneus, 5
Prepontine cistern, 12
Primary fissure, 5
Pulvinar, 4
Putamen, 16, 17, 18, 35, 36, 38
Pyramid
    medullary, 9, 31

Q

Quadrigeminal plate cistern,
    6, 15

R

Red nucleus, 15, 33

S

Sagittal sinus, 6, 16, 19, 20, 21,
    24, 25, 27, 38, 41, 44
Semicircular canal, 17, 32
Septum pellucidum, 6, 18, 36,
    49

Sigmoid sinus, 26
Sphenoid bone, 10
Straight sinus, 6, 18, 25, 27
Substantia nigra, 15, 32
Subthalamic nucleus, 33
Sulcus
    calcarine, 5, 17, 25, 27, 28
    central, 22
    cingulate, 5, 22, 31, 36
    inferior frontal, 42
    occipitotemporal, 33
    olfactory, 41, 42
    orbital, 15
    parietooccipital, 4, 5, 19, 25
    postcentral, 20
    post-olivary, 9
    precentral, 20, 21
    superior frontal, 21, 42, 43
Superior cerebellar artery, 56,
        60, 61
Superior colliculus, 30, 31, 53
Superior oblique muscle, 43
Superior rectus muscle, 43
Superior sagittal sinus, *See
        Sagittal sinus*
Suprachiasmatic recess, 51
Suprasellar cistern, 48
Sylvian fissure, 2, 19, 33, 36, 38

T

Temporal gyrus
    middle, 34
    superior, 34

Temporal lobe, 2, 12, 39
Tentorium, 2, 25, 29
Thalamus, 4, 16, 17, 31, 33,
        34
Third ventricle, 16, 32, 35, 48,
        49, 50
Torcular herophili, 14, 24
Transverse sinus, 12, 24, 25,
        26, 27
Trigeminal nerve, 11, 32, 33,
        34, 50, 51, 52
Trochlear nerve, 31
Tuber, 5

U

Uncinate fasciculus, 36
Uncus, 14
Uvula, 11, 28

V

Vein of Galen, 6, 30
Vermis, 26
Vertebral artery, 8, 33, 59
Vestibule, 32

W

White matter
    cerebellar, 27
    frontal, 22